The Big Short

MW00961314

by Michael Lewis

: This is a quick read summary based on the novel
"The Big Short"
by Michael Lewis

Note to Readers:

This is a Summary & Analysis of The Big Short by Michael Lewis. You are encouraged to buy the full version.

TABLE OF CONTENTS

OVERVIEW

This review of <u>The Big Short: Inside the Doomsday Machine</u> by Michael Lewis provides a chapter by chapter detailed summary followed by an analysis and critique of the strengths and weaknesses of the book.

The main theme explored in the book is how corruption and greed in Wall Street caused the crash of the subprime mortgage market in 2008. Despite being completely preventable, the big firms in Wall Street chose to ignore the oncoming fall in favor of making money. Michael Lewis introduces characters—men outside of the Wall Street machine—who foresaw the crisis and, through several different techniques, were able to predict how and when the market would fall. Lewis portrays these men—Steve Eisman, Mike Burry, Charlie Ledley, and Jamie Mai—as the underdogs, who were able to understand and act upon the obvious weaknesses in the subprime market. Lewis's overall point is to demonstrate how the Wall Street firms were manipulating the market. They used loans to cash in on the desperation of middle-to-lower class Americans, and then ultimately relied on the government to bail them out when the loans were defaulted.

Using anecdotes and interviews from the men who were involved first-hand, the author makes the case that Wall Street, and how they conducted business in regards to the subprime mortgage market, is truly corrupt beyond repair, and the men he profiles in this novel were trying to make the best out of a bad situation. By having the words from the sources themselves, this demonstrates Lewis's search for the truth behind what actually happened. Ultimately, we as an audience can not be sure if the intentions of these underdogs were truly good, but Lewis does an admirable job presenting as many sides to the story as possible.

The central thesis of the work is that the subprime mortgage crisis was caused by Wall Street firms pushing fraudulent loans upon middle-to-lower class Americans that they would essentially not be able to afford. Several people outside of Wall

Street were able to predict a crash in the market when these loans would be defaulted on, and bought insurance to bet against the market (essentially, buying short). Over a time period from roughly 2005-2008, the market crashed and huge banks and firms lost billions of dollars, filed for bankruptcy, or were bailed out by the government. These men, the characters of Lewis's novel, were able to bet against the loans and made huge amounts of money, but it was not quite an easy journey.

Michael Lewis is a non-fiction author and financial journalist. He has written several novels—notably *Liar's Poker* in 1989, *Moneyball* in 2003, and *The Blind Side* in 2006. Born in New Orleans, he attended Princeton University, receiving a BA degree in Art History. After attending London School of Economics and receiving his masters there, he was hired by Salomon Brothers where he experienced much about what he wrote about in *Liar's Poker*. He is currently married, with three children and lives in Berkeley, California.

SUMMARY
PROLOGUE: POLTERGEIST

Michael Lewis begins his tale of the remarkable—and strange—men who predicted the immense fall of the housing market by immediately exposing himself as the exact opposite type of person from them. He explains to the reader that he has no background in accounting, business, or money managing. Any success he has had with his previous book *Liar's Poker*, an account of his time working at Salomon Brothers in 1985, has been luck. That book had primarily been about the bond market and how that company, among many others in Wall Street, was making money off of selling and moving around the growing debt in America. Feeling like an outsider in the company, he left in 1988 and wrote the book as a period piece about finances in the 1980s. His wish was to appall America by exposing the very real money monsters such as CEO of Salomon Brothers, John Gutfreund, and Salomon's mortgage bond trader Howie Rubin. His message, however, was lost upon a materialistic America, who read his expose-esque novel as a how-to manual to succeeding in Wall Street.

While he did not succeed in his discrediting of the Wall Street money machine, he does introduce someone who came close: Meredith Whitney. Lewis introduces Whitney as an analyst of financial firms who worked for Oppenheimer and Co.. On October 31, 2007, she predicted that one of the biggest financial institutions—Citigroup—had been mismanaging their affairs and would likely go bankrupt. This one speculation turned the market upside down and caused their stocks to plummet. A virtual nobody in the business world managed with one word to cut eight percent off the Citigroup shares, forced CEO Chuck Prince to resign, and caused Citigroup to cut its dividend two weeks later. This had been the type of reaction Lewis had been hoping for with his first book. Her message is the same as his: Wall Street is not necessarily corrupt so much as they are simply stupid. Their jobs are to manage money, but they cannot seem to manage their own.

In March 2008, Lewis calls Whitney just as he is waiting for financial giant Bear Sterns to fall. He wants to discuss with her if this would be the moment that Wall Street would be brought down to reality once and for all. Before the call, Lewis explains reading an article in the news about a man, a small-time hedge fund manager named John Paulson, who had made $4 billion by betting against subprime mortgage bonds from huge Wall Street investment banks like Citigroup. His question for Whitney has now changed: who else had anticipated this subprime mortgage crash and who else stood to benefit from the fall of investment bank giants? In their conversation, Whitney gives him a list of six names or so of people she had personally advised or known about, including John Paulson and the man who begins Lewis's book: Steve Eisman.

CHAPTER 1: A SECRET ORIGIN STORY

Lewis begins his story about this remarkable cast of characters with the biggest character of them all: Steve Eisman. Eisman had grown up in New York City, graduated from the University of Pennsylvania magna cum laude, and graduated with honors from Harvard Law School. By 1991, Eisman finds himself a corporate lawyer with no sense of enjoyment for what he does. His parents encourage him to become an equity analyst as a means to learn about Wall Street, and that is where he begins his journey into the financial world: by working for people who shape the public's opinion about public companies.

Eisman is particularly talented at this as he is a proponent for breaking out from popular opinion and loves to make a lot of noise. Less than a year into his job, in December of 1991, a subprime mortgage lender named Aames Financial goes public. Eisman's company, Oppenheimer and Co., is looking for someone who knows about the mortgage business in hopes that they could use them as a liaison to be hired by this new company. Eisman has previous experience proofreading—and misunderstanding—documents for a deal with a small time mortgage company and is duly appointed the lead analyst for Aames Financial. The problem with Aames Financial, he finds, is that their intentions are to extend loans to lower middle class and poor Americans through a unique type of loan called "subprime mortgages."

After having secured this position, Eisman begins to stretch his muscles and quickly established himself as one of the few analysts at his company whose opinion stirs the markets. He proves this with another company called Lomas Financial Corp, who, despite their efforts to push good press, fall into bankruptcy a few months after Eisman publicly declares a sell rating on their stock. This demonstrates how powerful Eisman's words and opinions are becoming to the public.

Lewis goes in depth about the love/hate relationship people had with Eisman. He provides many colorful examples of his personality quirks such as leaving in the middle of a huge corporate meeting to answer his cell phone (only to never return) and offending a Japanese business man with his frankness. In interviews with Eisman, Lewis demonstrates how unclearly Eisman sees himself, and is actually surprised at how people respond to him. Lewis provides two theories about his behavior (suggested by the people who know him best): one, he is much more interested in what is going on in his own head than what is outside of it, and two, he actually lives with a dichotomy in his personality. He is described as both the person who would do anything for another human being, selfless to the point of stupidity, but he also having a craving to know and understand the internal contradictions behind human behavior. He is both an optimist and pessimist.

The author then sets the scene for the crisis to come. He begins with the creation of the mortgage bond market and how it extends Wall Street into the debts of ordinary Americans.

Before long, big time money making firms are finding fuel from the debts of the least-solvent portion of the American population. No one truly expected that mortgage bonds could be such a money maker for banks as they are not the quickest and most guaranteed form of accumulating the in-debt public's money. This is because often borrowers repay their loans after interest rates have fallen and are able to refinance at a cheaper price. Loaners solved this as they learned to pool together the home loans and carve up the payments into "tranches."

Lewis explains that in the 1980's, the worse thing for an investor would be if a bond was repaid too quickly because the loans carry a government guarantee that pays off a homeowner's debts if they default. Pretty soon, lenders began selling mortgage bonds that did not qualify for these government guarantees in order to be able to extend credit to less and less creditworthy homeowners, cashing out equity on the houses they owned. This ruins the safety of tranches for investors by allowing lower-middle-class Americans to pay lower interest rates on their debts. Eisman, in the midst of his job as analyst crusader, begins to take many of these subprime companies public, naively believing that they really are helping the consumer by taking them out of high interest rate credit card debt and putting them into low interest rate mortgage debt. It takes something big for him to realize the error of his ways.

Here, Lewis introduces Vincent Daniel, a naturally suspicious man from Queens, New York, and highlights the differences between Daniel and Eisman, right up until describing how they meet. In giving his background on Daniel, Lewis describes how he worked as a junior accountant auditing Salomon Brothers. There, his eyes were opened to the questionable books they kept and how little any of accountants could explain about what was actually going on. Realizing that it was futile to try to audit a giant Wall Street firm in aims of determining if it was making or losing money, Daniel quits. His resume finds itself in the hands of Eisman at Oppenheimer and Co.. Eisman happens to be looking for someone to help him understand the increasingly complicated accounting used by subprime mortgages and Daniel seems to fit the bill. During their phone interview, Eisman puts Daniel on hold, yet never answers back. It is not until a few months later that Daniel is given the job and later finds out that the interruption was caused by a phone call informing Eisman that his newborn son Max had died. Everyone in Eisman's life notices a distinct change in him: while he previously went through life thinking himself protected and safe, this accident (their night nurse rolled on top of the son and smothered him in her sleep) showed him that anything could happen.

After this, Eisman is more disposed to be outspoken and even rude about some of the subprime mortgage companies. While his initial bashing of the less viable companies seems to be taken with a grain of salt, his damning of the industry becomes so heightened that even his employer begins to find it financially counterproductive. Eisman wants to write a report that will shut down the entire system, and challenges Daniel to help him find his ammunition. At this time, a rating system called Moody's has just offered to sell information about subprime mortgage loans. Daniel is tasked with going in and figuring it all out. Here, he finds that companies seem to only disclose what they earned and completely ignore the delinquency rate of the home loans they sold.

Another disturbing thing that Daniel notices is that certain loans, particularly ones on mobile homes, are being prepaid at very quick rates. He discovers that the prepayments are so high because they were involuntary, meaning defaulted. Essentially what is happening is that these mobile home buyers are defaulting on their loans, having their homes repossessed, and the people who lent them the money are receiving fractions of the original loans. The people are duped into buying these loans because even though the interest rates are not high enough to justify this risk, it was obvious that they are attempting to make poor people feel wealthy by giving them cheap loans. After six months of sifting through this information, Daniel informs Eisman that these subprime mortgage companies are covering their lack of any real earnings by growing their mortgage loans rapidly and using creative accounting.

Eisman writes his report. In it, he provides the actual difference in numbers between what the companies are reporting and what they are actually earning. The companies lose it. They claim his data is incorrect, that he did not give them a fair warning for them to defend themselves, and that he has violated the Wall Street code. This report, written in September 1997, has a ripple effect and causes several companies, including a hedge fund called Long-Term Capital Management, to go bankrupt. Despite his crusading, Eisman tires of his work at Oppenheimer and quits to work at a hedge fund called Chilton Investment. Here, he hopes he can get out of being an analyst, trust his own judgements, and learn how to manage money. The company has other ideas and keeps him in his previous role of analyzing companies for actual money managers. Despite hating his job, Eisman fortuitously learns what is really going on inside the consumer loan market.

In early 2002, he receives consumer lending giant Household Finance Corporation's new sales document that offers a new type of home equity loan. Despite the bust in several similar companies and Americans uneager to take on any new debts, Household is booming in their loans. Their greatest source of growth is with second mortgages, offering a fifteen-year, fixed-rate loan that is presented as a thirty-year loan. In packaging it this way, their sales pitch dishonestly claims a interest rate of 7 percent, when in fact is closer to 12.5. Eisman focuses his sole attention on crusading against Household's tactics. He contacts every form of media that he can, even badgering the office of the attorney general of state. Despite his best efforts, not even the government will intervene and Household goes on to sell itself and its portfolio for $15.5 billion. Eisman comes to the realization that the subprime mortgage system is not looking out for the little guy.

As he is denied the chance to manage money, Eisman quits and attempts to start his own hedge fund called FrontPoint Partners. In 2004, Morgan Stanley, their umbrella company, allows him to set up a fund that focuses entirely on financial companies with the stipulation that he raise his own money for it. He travels across the United States and Europe searching for investors. Only one, an insurance company, gives him $50 million, which is not quite enough to sustain an equity fund. Lewis explains that while Eisman could not attract money, he does attract people. Adding to his team of crusaders is Daniel, Porter Collins, who he worked with at Chilton Investment, and Danny Moses, a salesman at Oppenheimer and Co..

By the time this group forms in 2005, subprime lending is becoming increasingly murky. In 2000, there is $130 billion in subprime mortgage lending and by 2005 it booms to $625 billion. Even the terms are changing. In 1996, 65% of the loans were at a fixed-rate, insuring that the consumer knew how much they would need to pay each month. Yet, by 2005, 75% of these same loans are at a floating-rate, leaving the consumer completely at mercy to the whims of these companies. These companies are getting so good at finding new ways to siphon more money from the middle to lower classes that all the largest Wall Street investment banks join in on the subprime game. Eisman has an epiphany moment after his first year of running his own company: he had been so focused on choosing the right stocks, that he was completely ignoring that the stocks were dependent on the bonds. These financial companies that run those bonds are becoming increasingly exposed to the subprime mortgage market.

Chapter 2: In the Land of the Blind

Lewis begins chapter two by introducing another man in his cast of characters: Michael Burry. He describes Burry as single handedly teaching himself how to borrow and lend money in the bond market. To Burry, it is an obsession of sorts, an aspect of his personality that would be prevalent throughout the novel. Burry is particularly interested in how subprime mortgage bonds work. He finds that individual loans are built up into towers, with the top floors having the lowest interest rate, and thus receiving their money back first, and the lower floors suffering the highest risk by getting their money back last. Because of this, they have the highest interests rates. Essentially, investors can choose which floor they want to invest in. Michael Burry studies these not to invest, but to learn, in particular, how he can short the mortgage bonds. In the beginning of 2005, he scans hundreds of loans and notices that there is a clear decline in lending standards from as early as 2004. Burry sees this bottom as the "interest-only negative-amortizing adjustable-rate subprime mortgage." With these loans, the home buyer is given the option to not pay anything and roll over the interest they have into a higher principal balance. Obviously, this is meant for a homeowner with little to no income. Burry sets about figuring out why a money lender would want a loan like this at all.

The more Burry investigates, the more he discovers that lenders have been degrading their standards to grow loan volumes. Now there is a snag in his plan: because the lenders are selling their mortgages to big banks, who in turn package them and sell them off to buyers, Burry could not sell them short as he intended. Instead, he buys credit default swaps, and purchases insurance on companies he thinks would suffer if there was a real estate downturn. Still not satisfied, Burry wants a stronger bet against the market, and he finds it in the two-year "teaser" rates that many mortgages offer. Many that were sold in 2005 have a fixed rate as low as 6 percent, but after that time, they would balloon to 11 percent and upwards, resulting in a wave of defaults. Burry wants to bet on these defaults, but discovers that there is not a way—yet. After calling several of the top banks he believes would survive such a downfall, he discovers that most have no idea what he is talking about, and others want to ignore the problem altogether.

Here, Lewis interjects a bit more background on Burry. When he was two years old, he developed a rare type of cancer and a resulting operation caused the loss of his left eye. For all of his life he felt his differences in behavior, personality, and how he saw the world were a result of seeing with only one eye. People were often frustrated by his lack of social skills or verbal signal recognition, but Burry and his family always chalked it up to his glass eye. Burry often portrayed obsessiveness towards whatever task or interest that was at hand, and preferred activities that involved very little social interaction. In 1998, during his residency in neurology at Stanford Hospital, he told his superiors that he had spent the past two nights in a row completely rebuilding his personal computer, all while working fourteen hour shifts. His superiors requested a psychiatrist evaluation which diagnosed him as bipolar. Burry was positive this was wrong. Medicine, never having been particularly interesting to him, now disgusted and frustrated him and so he quits.

Thinking back to his childhood, when his father would show him the stock tables at the back of the newspaper and tell him never to trust the crooked market, Burry decides to focus his energies on making sense of the illogical market. Burry becomes a "value investor," essentially teaching himself how to do it. Like other ventures in his life, such as high school, college, and medical school, he works alone, educating himself on how to become a financial expert.

His journey in to Wall Street begins one night in November 1996 as he is on a cardiology rotation at St. Thomas Hospital. On a hospital computer, he discovers a website called techstocks.com where he creates a thread about value investing and how to invest in the real world. Little by little he begins a discussion and shares his own tips on how to manage money. After a while, he gets the sense that people have been taking his advice and making money from it. From this, he starts his own blog, working on it between sixteen hour shifts at the hospital. His advice becomes so popular that even people from big time firms like Fidelity and Morgan Stanley are visiting his blog regularly. He realizes the full impact he is having when one time he writes a very negative post about a company named Vanguard, and their lawyers send him a cease and desist order almost immediately.

By this time, Burry had been experiencing a lot of big life events: he had moved back to San Jose, his father died, he was remarried, and he had been (mis)diagnosed as bipolar. He shuts down his website and decides to quit medicine to become a full time money manager. Using the money his father left him, as well as bits from his family, he starts Scion Capital. Potential investors in his company are issued a memo that he would not be accepting anyone worth less than $15 million: an interesting irony as this would exclude all the people he knew, including himself.

His first investor is Gotham Capital, who tells him that their founder Joel Greenblatt had been making money off of Burry's blog for years and they want to continue to do so. They fly him out to New York and they meet—him in a t-shirt and sweatpants—and offer him a million dollars for a quarter of his fund. Shortly after this, Burry receives a call from White Mountains, an insurance holding company, who heard about the Gotham deal and offers him $600,000 for a smaller piece of his fund and another $10 million to invest in his company. He had started his company with little more than a million dollars and by 2004 he was managing $600 million and turning away investors.

Part of what made Burry so successful, Lewis explains, is that he understands that people respond to negative incentives. Lewis gives examples of insurance reimbursements for appendectomies creating a boom in the operations, as well as the dangers of a certain ophthalmology procedure leading to the creation of Lasik. Understanding this, Burry makes sure that he has the right incentives in his business. Doing nothing more than buying common stocks and reading financial statements, Burry turns his shrewd investments into a fund up 242 percent from when it opened. His specialty is what he calls "ick" investments, something he explains means investing in a stock that creates a first reaction of "ick." One example is the Avant! Corporation and how Burry reads that they were accused of stealing computer code. After doing some digging he realizes the potential, that is, if he can stomach short term loses and his investors freaking out about negative publicity. He buys shares in June 2001 at $12 a share and as the company's dirty deeds hit the press, the stock falls all the way down to $2 a share, where Burry happily scoops them up. After becoming the single largest shareholder, he contacts the company and demands they make changes, and clean up their reputation. After four months of this, their stocks rise to $22 a share.

This practice of short-term loss to long-term gain is Burry's specialty, and he knows that this tactic makes investors nervous. So, he removes the possibility of them pulling out by only allowing them to invest for one to two full years. This gives him time to allow the market to adjust to what he knows it will do. Here, Lewis returns to the subprime mortgage bond market and 2005. The biggest concern of Burry's, at this point, is that the banks are not selling him the credit default swaps fast enough. He is sure that they, as well as the rest of the U.S. housing market, will realize the chaos to come and make things right (or at the very least, sense what he did and raise the prices).

Another concern of his is that he suspects that whoever sold him a credit default swap will one day owe him a lot of money, and there was a strong possibility that they might try to get out of it. So he goes to the International Swaps and Derivatives Association to draft a contract to guarantee this from happening. As the terms are being finalized in May 2005, Burry makes his first subprime mortgage deals from Deutsche Bank on six different bonds. He only seeks out the dodgiest pools of mortgages to buy insurance against and is surprised when Deutsche Bank does not question his choices. He is sure that they will catch on and adjust their prices, but instead even more banks begin to call him, offering him more of the worst mortgage bonds to choose from. In just a few weeks, he has purchased several hundred million dollars in credit default swaps from six different banks, none of whom seem to care that he is choosing the worst loans. Goldman Sachs even asks him in June 2005 if he wants to increase his trade size from $10 million at a time to $100 million. Burry is happy to accept.

It is absolutely incredible to him that there are people out there willing to sell him insane amounts of cheap insurance on bonds that are ticking time bombs. This gives him the idea to start a fund that focuses entirely on doing what he had been spending all of his time and money doing anyways. He creates a new business and calls this insurance purchasing fund "Milton's Opus." While his investors in this company are happy to let him pick their stocks, they are less than enthusiastic in believing he can foresee huge trends in the subprime mortgage market and their lack of support causes the company to die pretty quickly.

In October of 2005, Burry decides to tell the truth of what he had been doing with their money to his investors at Scion: they own more than a billion dollars in credit default swaps in the subprime mortgage bond market. Most investors are not very pleased. Lewis describes them as being macro-thinkers, people who could not believe that one man could possibly have a deeper understanding of global trends and forces than any of the big banks or the market itself. When it came down to it, they appreciated his spirit, but lost interest when it not only did not earn them money, but tied their money up in an area they had no clue about.

Just as his investors are becoming uneasy, Burry receives a call from a trader at Goldman Sachs, asking him why he is buying swaps from such specific groupings of the subprime bonds. Other companies want to learn how to trade like Scion. As the market begins to unravel, Burry receives an email from the head of subprime mortgages at Deutsche Bank, Greg Lippmann. He wants to buy back the first six credit default swaps that Burry purchased in May. Figuring that the $60 million sum is small compared to his now rich portfolio, as well as wanting to cut ties with Deutsche altogether, he agrees. It is not until they offer to buy more of his other swaps that he questions how they knew about it all in the first place. This question grows larger as he receives calls from more and more big time banks like Goldman Sachs, Bank of America, and Morgan Stanley.

At this point, the loans that were set to go off in two years are finally doing so and everyone is catching on. *The New York Times* releases an article about this in November and Burry understands that all these changes are occurring because the cat is out of the bag.

CHAPTER 3: "HOW CAN A GUY WHO CAN'T SPEAK ENGLISH LIE?"

Lewis begins this chapter by focusing on the introduction of Greg Lippmann (the subprime manager at Deutsch Bank) to Steve Eisman and his FrontPoint crew in February 2006. The general consensus at this meeting is not to trust Lippmann, who is shown to be a sort of fast-talking conman. He is described as being obviously self-interested and self-promotional. In general, the bond market is not subject to the same kind of regulation as the stock market, and bond salesman can essentially say and do anything they want to close a deal. Lippmann is famous for playing on the fear and ignorance of his customers to sell his bonds. The FrontPoint men know this and are inherently, and rightfully, suspicious. Lippmann approaches Eisman and his men with what he deems his own idea on how to bet against the subprime mortgage bond market, which essentially is the same idea that Mike Burry has been utilizing this whole time.

Eisman, ever the crusader against big Wall Street, is interested. He no longer needs to worry about time, because he can now clearly see (rather than guess) when the market will crash, and even further, he does not need to put up a lot of cash up front. What really seals the deal for Eisman is Lippmann's associate, Eugene Xu, a national math competition winner from China who is responsible for all of the hard data and numbers in Lippmann's presentation. They figure that he must be telling the truth because not only do numbers not lie, but: "How can a guy who can't speak English lie?" Lippmann plays on all of Eisman's possible vanities—he might become so rich he can buy the Dodgers, movie stars will be more attracted to him, etc. Eisman, of course, is not interested in any of this. He is intrigued by the proposition, but only wants to know how a credit default swap works and why Lippmann is betting against his own bank. While Eisman is more curious than suspicious, his fellow FrontPoint men are not impressed.

Lewis shifts back to Burry and where he stands at this moment. At this time, Burry is curious as to who is on the other side of these deals, unknowingly going against a triple-A rated insurance company called American International Group, Inc. (AIG). This company set the model for all future insurance companies, and essentially created and developed the idea of credit default swaps that Burry was cashing in on. Working with AIG, the bank Goldman Sachs had spent years fiddling with the business of subprime mortgages and over time developed a security that was so cloudy and unintelligible that no investor or rating agency could make heads or tails of it. This is the beginning of the collateralized debt obligation (CDO) which is the main way that banks laundered credit for lower to middle class Americans. It literally turned lead into gold for the Wall Street banks.

Lewis reveals that these banks are using CDOs to generate more money, simply from nowhere: and that is why they need people like Mike Burry and Eisman to buy $10 million in credit default swaps. The bank takes these hundreds of different triple-B bonds and packages them into synthetic CDOs. They then take them to rating agencies with the bank's own rating system and make them look like triple-A bonds. They do not need billion dollar loans, they just need ones that look like billion dollar loans, to be able to sell them to an unknowing investor. In this way, Mike Burry is buying insurance that is being run through this system, without knowing. All the banks know how unethical this is, but no one stands up, and some banks, like Deutsch, want to cash in big from it.

Lippmann's bosses at Deutsch want him to be the stand-in for Mike Burry and make a bet against the market. This way, he can take these swaps he made against his own bank and trade them with AIG in order to profit. Mike Burry realizes this profit too and wants desperately to trade in as well. AIG is more than willing, but he has a hard time finding investors: no one wants to bet against the subprime mortgage market no matter how poorly it was doing. Lippmann is also having difficulty getting people on board. He decides to offer people the opportunity to get out of their credit default swaps—for a hefty fee, of course—promising that they will make a fortune. People still see through his motives so he is forced to take another tact: he wants to kill the new market. AIG is still the only other person on the other side of the market and so in 2005, Lippmann flies to London to try and stop them from buying bonds, thus insuring that the entire subprime mortgage bond market will collapse.

CHAPTER 4: HOW TO HARVEST A MIGRANT WORKER

Lippmann's meeting awakens AIG to how the banks have been playing them for fools, but he is not the first person to be alerted to this. One of their employees, Gene Park, begins to notice that the quality of the subprime mortgages has become very low. He realizes that the piles of consumer loans they are insuring are containing more and more of these mortgages and sees the possibility that AIG may not be able to handle it when consumers begin to default on their loans. When he takes this to his superiors, they merely scream at him that he had no idea what is going on. Park begins an ongoing feud with his boss, Joe Cassano who is described by Lewis as knowingly creating a deeper hole for AIG, regardless of future consequences. After a lot of prodding, and meeting with several huge banks who all claim that the market could never fall, Cassano changes his mind and agrees that AIG should not insure any more of these deals.

On Lippmann's side, he believes it is his presentation in London that does it, but no matter the reasons, AIG is finished insuring these questionable loans. Lippmann then goes on a search to find stock market investors that might be scared into joining him in his hedge fund. This is when he finds Eisman and the FrontPoint crew. He is sure that Eisman will join in the bet against the subprime market, but surprisingly, he does not agree right away. It is not until several months later that FrontPoint calls him in to explain his idea once more. This is because Standard & Poor changes it's model to rate subprime mortgage bonds and the price of insuring bonds falls drastically.

While Burry is busy betting on pools of loans with high concentrations of the kinds of structures he believes would ultimately fail, Eisman and his crew are focused on the people doing the borrowing and lending. They call Wall Street traders and asked for "menus" of the subprime bonds, trying to find the most rotten so they can buy the smartest insurance. Lewis describes these bonds as having similar characteristics, like being from the same states, coming from the same dubious lenders, and having a higher than average possibility of being fraudulent. They witness a growing pattern in lending to the very poor and immigrants, mostly due to how loan packagers pool FICO scores of their loanees, rather than examining them individually. By having no difference between people with little to no credit (like immigrants) and those with a lengthy credit history, the FICO scores are virtually the same.

Eisman's goal, at this point, is to learn as much as he can about how the rating agencies have been tricked. He and his team spend months trying to find the most overrated bonds in the market. During this time, they buy their first credit default swaps from Lippmann. Daniel and Moses at FrontPoint fly to Orlando for a subprime mortgage bond conference called ABS East. Here, they come face to face with the rating agencies and Lippmann gets them personal meetings under the condition that they tell them they are betting for—not against—their bonds. Everything they learn at the conference is worse than they expect. One woman, from the rating agency Moody's, tells them that even though her job is to evaluate subprime mortgage bonds, her bosses do not allow her to downgrade the ones that she knows should be. Daniel reports back to Eisman that the industry is so much more corrupt than they originally thought. Despite their shock at how deep the immorality runs, Lewis hints at a much bigger conference to come, with larger and worse players, being held in Las Vegas.

CHAPTER 5: ACCIDENTAL CAPITALISTS

By the fall of 2006, Lippmann has brought his idea to nearly 250 investors privately and hundreds more through conferences at Deutsche Bank. This is a point that Lewis makes clear: people are aware what is going to happen. Yet, only a hundred or so actually take Lippmann's advice and buy insurance (mostly to hedge against the bet against themselves), and only a dozen make a straightforward bet against the market. Lewis highlights how extraordinary this is as it is incredibly clear how foreseeable the fall is, yet people still did not want to see it.

One man who succeeds where Burry fails in creating his own firm is John Paulson. He is able to raise billions of dollars from investors in exchange for insurance on their real estate portfolios. Another unusual character is Charlie Ledley, who usually bets on whatever he believes Wall Street thought was least likely to happen. He reads Lippmann's proposal in September 2006 and thinks it is too good to be true. Along with his partner Jamie Mai, he opens a money management firm out of a shed behind their friend's house in Berkeley, California. They call their business Cornwall Capital Management and their aim is to find market inefficiency across the global market. Their first big lesson comes from Capital One, where they capitalize on the stock price's inability to incorporate corruption into its model and are able to buy cheap long-term stock options. This becomes their main technique. They do the same with a distressed European cable company called United Pan-European Cable, buying $500,000 options and turning them in to a $5 million profit. They eventually come up with a term for what they are doing: event-driven investing.

Lewis explains that they are so successful with this technique because the market underestimates any extreme moves in prices: it is essentially short-sighted. Even further, the price of stock is reflective of its past volatility, so it does not really reflect what might come but rather what has happened. Using this knowledge, Cornwall is running $12 million of their own money after only two years of opening. The problem they now face is that big time banks only see them as a "garage band hedge fund" and do not allow them to buy long options on their stocks—something that could drastically change their profits. Somehow, they are able to persuade Deutsche Bank to accept Cornwall on an "institutional platform." They meet with a team from the bank to see if they were worthy of the distinction. From this very awkward meeting, they finally get their ISDA license and are given the ability to trade with the big guys.

Lippmann's sales pitch reaches Cornwall and the men are intrigued. They had never bought or sold mortgage bonds before, but they can see the financial benefit of the trade. Even better, they realize that they are being given a cheap opportunity to have front row tickets to the inevitable drama of the fall of the market. Coming into the trades so late in the game is actually beneficial for them, as it allows them to be able to move much faster than Burry was able to as they did not really have to do any of the same initial research: it was already done for them. By January 2007, they own $110 million in credit default swaps and are prepared to witness a thrilling fallout when they are invited to go to a big annual subprime conference in Las Vegas.

CHAPTER 6: SPIDER-MAN AT THE VENETIAN

This chapter focuses mainly on the big conference for subprime mortgages in Las Vegas, Nevada, and it is here that most of the cast of characters Lewis has been introducing converge. He begins with Eisman and his crew at FrontPoint. Eisman, not knowing what to do, relies on Lippmann to help him with connections. Lippmann had recently encountered a new problem in that house prices were falling, people were defaulting quickly, and yet the subprime bonds, as well as the prices to insure them, were staying steady. This causes a lot of investors he had been promising would benefit from the defaults to lose faith in his plan. So, to remedy this, he invites many of his investors to a dinner at the Okada restaurant in Vegas. Seated around four different hibachi islands, he carefully plants at least one hedge fund manager that was persuaded to short the bonds. The rest of the table is filled out with investors who are long on those bonds. Lippmann's hope is that the hedge fund people will see the other investors as stupid and not worry so much about the lack of current success in his pitch.

Eisman in particular is seated next to someone named Wing Chau, a man who controls $15 billion in triple B-rated CDOs. Chau, very pleased with himself, explains that he is passing all the risk of the home loans onto bigger investors who hired him. While under the guise of being a CDO expert, he is paying more attention to how to maximize the money earned from the CDOs than regulating them. Eisman is infuriated by this man, as was Lippmann's plan. Even further, Chau reveals how happy he is that people like Eisman are shorting his market. The more trades they do, the more product he gains and this hits Eisman like a truck. He finally realizes why the banks are so eager to accept their trades: the more he shorts, the more the banks are able to synthesize the worst CDOs and make money out of nothing.

After the meal, Eisman tells Lippmann that he wants to short everything that Chau is buying. Up to this point, he had only been shorting the swaps on subprime mortgages, but now he wanted to specifically go against Chau and buy swaps on Chau's CDOs.

Meanwhile, the men with Cornwall are frantically trying to understand their place at the conference. They try desperately to meet people, sneaking up on speakers at podiums right after their speeches. The more people they listen to, the more they realize that the long shot they have taken in making $100 million in credit default swaps on the unlikely event that the double A rated bonds would collapse is actually the most likely event to occur. At the opening ceremony for the conference, they hear a speech made by John Devaney, who runs United Capital Markets, a hedge fund that specifically invests in subprime mortgages. Devaney, clearly still inebriated from the night before, rants about the state of the market. The more they listen to his speech, the more spooked the Cornwall men become as the fall feels closer than ever before.

Going back to Eisman, Lewis explains that Deutsche Bank hires their CDO salesman Ryan Stark to keep an eye on Eisman to insure he is not causing any trouble. Eisman, of course, is not there to buy bonds and certainly does not care to pretend. Lewis describes Eisman's attitude here by explaining that he sees himself as "Spider-Man," a champion of the underdog. One morning during a speech given by the CEO of Option One, Eisman proves his crusade by publicly arguing with the CEO during his speech. It is clear to Lewis that it is here in Vegas that Eisman's attitude towards the bond market hardens. They go in wondering what the bond market knows that they do not and then leave realizing that these employees very likely should be fired or in jail because they either know exactly what they are doing, or are completely delusional. Eisman and his team started their Vegas trip with a short of

$300 million and leave with $550 million in new bets against CDOs.

CHAPTER 7: THE GREAT TREASURE HUNT

Ledley and Hockett from Cornwall return from Vegas convinced that the financial system has lost its mind. The day after market insiders return to their desks, the market cracks. The Cornwall men are terrified that they discovered this trade a moment too late and on February 16, 2007 they buy $10 million in credit default swaps on a CDO called Gulfstream. Five days later the market begins publicly trading on these CDOs and the Cornwall group receive a whirlwind of emails from people at Morgan Stanley and Deutsche Bank, telling them to ignore the prices on these new CDOs, they will not change the value of the ones they just purchased. When they try to call Morgan Stanley the next day to buy more insurance, the company will not let them. They changed their minds virtually overnight and from then on, Cornwall no longer works with them.

It seems to Cornwall Capital that even though the CDO market is still going, the big Wall Street banks had caught on and have no more use for investors. Cornwall is trying desperately to buy more swaps, but no one will sell. Out of nowhere, between February and June of 2007, several huge firms create and sell $50 billion in new CDOs. It is clear to the Cornwall group that Wall Street did this in an effort to raise the price of the CDOs and dump the losses on the consumer: making a last few billion dollars off of the corrupted market. Cornwall attempts to alert the media, and even contacts the SEC, but no one believes them.

Then, Cornwall faces a huge problem. On June 14, 2007, their main trading company, Bear Stearns, publicly declares that it had lost money on their subprime mortgage bets and dumps $3.8 billion worth of bets before closing their fund. Cornwall had bought 70% of their swaps from Bear Stearns and now it is likely that they are not going to pay off their debts. Fortunately, the men at Cornwall had also purchased $105 million in swaps on Bear Stearns back in March—effectively betting on the collapse of the firm. However, they did this deal with another big firm—HSBC in Britain—and this really just places their risk into the hands of another bank.

Lewis turns his attention again to Eisman and his reaction to the news that HSBC and Merrill Lynch are publicly declaring their losses in the subprime mortgage market between February and July of 2007. Because they are still declaring profitable quarters, despite the losses, Eisman begins to suspect that there is more going on. He is sure that it is not that they are lying, so much that they truly do not believe that the subprime market is a problem for them. He sets his team out to conduct a "Great Treasure Hunt" to figure out if there are firms out there that are somehow also betting against the subprime bonds—but ultimately, they discover nothing.

In July 2007, FrontPoint holds a small conference with their investors. They outright share what they know about the subprime market and what is likely about to happen. He explains everything that he knows about the bonds, the credit default swaps, and CDOs. Finally, Eisman tells his investors that he is expecting the market to lose up to $300 billion. An editor from Grant's Interest Rate Observer, Jim Grant, had been prophesizing this doom ever since the mid-1980s when the debt cycle began. He investigated these CDOs and wrote a series of pieces on them in early 2007 suggesting that the agencies were rating them without actually checking or knowing what was inside of them. This confirms Eisman's theory about the financial world and gives him the courage to share with his investors that he knows that he is on the right track.

CHAPTER 8: THE LONG QUIET

It is now February 2007 and the subprime loans are defaulting as expected, yet Mike Burry's investors are growing impatient. They mistrust that he will provide the profits he promised, but Burry knows that it is only a matter of time until the teaser rate period is over. Lewis explains that this is a very lonely period of time for Burry. In order to keep placing bets against the bonds, he is forced to fire half his staff and nearly everyone he works with mistrusts him. Even further, he and his wife have their son tested by a child psychologist to discover that he has Asperger's, which they realize—after doing extensive research and reading on the syndrome—Burry also has. He feels this explains a lot about his life and personality, and begins to work with a psychologist to help him sort out the effects of the syndrome. He keeps this information from his investors, feeling that this aspect of his personality is likely why he has been so successful.

Unusually, as the loans began to reach their teaser rate end period, the price of insuring the loans is dropping. By the middle of 2006, money managers begin calling Burry asking for help on how to make the same bets he is making. Even though success is on the horizon, Burry is miserable. His investors hound him for reports: what he is spending their money on, why he chooses certain loans, and why they have not been able to cash in yet. This is not how Burry works, and he believes he had made himself clear about that when he started his business. Burry is forced to send a letter to his investors stating that he is locking up between 50-55 percent of their money and provides a quarterly report, showing where it will be going. Immediately there is backlash. His partners at Gotham Capital threaten to sue him, and several others begin to organize themselves into a legal fight. This isolates him even further.

In January 2007, just as the others are meeting in Las Vegas, Burry sits down with his investors to explain how even though the S&P rose 10% that year, he has lost 18.4%. He attempts to mitigate this by reminding them that the credit default swaps are about to cash in soon enough as three of the big mortgage originators had failed in just the past two months. But his investors see him as a villain and routinely leak his quarterly letters to the press to be picked apart.

But then something changes. On June 14, two of the subprime hedge funds owned by Bear Stearns falls and the publicly traded index of triple-B rated bonds falls by 20 percent. Goldman Sachs experiences a sort-of nervous breakdown and their bond saleswoman vanishes. Upon her return, as well as the return of representatives of several other head banks that mysteriously disappeared, she claims a "systems failure." More news of banks falling, or attempting to create fairer rates for the bonds and insurance makes Burry realize that this is the moment he has been waiting for. By the end of year, the defaults on loans have spiked to 37.7 percent, showing that more than a third of the borrowers have defaulted.

After this, Burry is reading in the paper about the genius of people (like John Paulson) who saw this coming, people who had come into the trade much later than he had. Even Greg Lippmann is credited for seeing this catastrophe ahead of time, and making huge sums of money from it. Burry receives no credit and no gratitude, especially from his investors.

CHAPTER 9: A DEATH OF INTEREST

In the second to last chapter, Lewis provides a little insight into why credit default swaps were created, from the voice of one of the men involved at the inception: Howie Hubler. Hubler, who ran Morgan Stanley's asset-backed bond trading, was put in charge of the firm's bets on subprime mortgages. For nearly a decade before the other groups were making bets in 2004, Hubler and his subprime mortgage desk were creating bonds and making money at a growing pace. As interest grew, they had to "warehouse" loans, and this put them at risk to falling prices between when the purchase of the loan was made and when they actually could sell the bonds. To protect them, one of Hubler's associates, Mike Edman, created the credit default swaps. He solved the problem by adding fine print in their contracts, specifying that Morgan Stanley was buying insurance on the last outstanding loan in the pool from the swap.

Using this idea, Hubler is able to acquire $2 billion worth of credit default swaps by early 2005. By the spring of that year, Hubler and his associates are sure that the policies will pay off, but it is around this time that Burry begins to buy his swaps, agitating their plan. Because of him, and Greg Lippmann at Deutsch Bank, Morgan Stanley is now forced to trade their credit default swaps openly and lose out on being the only fish in the pool. As incentive not to quit and open his own hedge fund, Morgan Stanley offers Hubler his own proprietary trading group called Global Proprietary Credit Group in which Hubler is allowed to keep some of the profits he earns in the company.

While the conference in Vegas is commencing, Hubler is selling swaps on roughly 16 billion dollars of CDOs. He is making the same bets on the same CDO tranches as the Cornwall Capital, FrontPoint, and Scion Capital men. One by one the banks abandon the subprime market: J.P. Morgan in the fall of 2006, Goldman Sachs after that (even betting against the market after getting out), and so on.

In early July, Morgan Stanley receives a call from Lippmann that the $4 billion in swaps that Hubler sold Deutsche Bank six months earlier is now in their favor: Morgan Stanley owes Deutsch $1.2 billion by the end of the day. This is what causes Hubler to back out. He does not want to take a full loss, so he insists that his CDOs are still worth more, and his superiors (also not wanting to declare a full loss) agree to send Deutsche over $600 million. Those same bonds continue to crash and Deutsche offers Morgan Stanley an exit to their trade. As he continues to decline, Hubler is finally forced to resign in October 2007, leaving behind losses as big as $9 billion—the largest trading loss in Wall Street history.

Finally, the moment all these men have been waiting for arrives: there are no more buyers of the subprime mortgage bonds. Shareholders bring a lawsuit to Bear Stearns on August 1, 2007, connecting them to the collapse of the subprime-based hedge funds. This alarms the Cornwall Capital men as most of their credit default swaps had been purchased from Bear Stearns. They realized that if somehow the market bounced back (say, the government bailed them out), they could lose a lot of money. The Cornwall group rushes to find a buyer of the insurance policies they had collected. UBS, a bank that had been begging them for months to purchase their insurance, takes these swaps off Cornwall's hands, suggesting that they do not imagine that a monolith such as Bear Stearns could fall.

In late August, Burry allows his investors to have their money back, and with twice as much as they had given him. By the end of that year alone, his $550 million profile had earned profits of more than $720 million.

CHAPTER 10: TWO MEN IN A BOAT

Lewis explains in his final chapter how Eisman's crusade against the subprime market is not so much about making money, but is nearly meant as an insult to the Wall Street goliaths that were trying to pull one over on middle-to-lower class Americans. His gamble against the market is his way to tell the people inside the big firms that they should have known better. His "Great Treasure Hunt" provides him a long list of companies that are exposed by these loans, and by March 2008, nearly every firm on his list has sold short their stocks.

The author reviews the two phases of how the market fell. First, AIG takes most of the risk of the market collapse, until the end of 2005 when they stop out of nowhere. They hope to stall the market by doing this, but Wall Street continues on, making more money than ever with their CDOs. This lead into the second phase where, over the course of two years, firms are creating between $200 and $400 billion in subprime-backed CDOs. By March 2008, around the time that the teaser-rates are over and people are completely defaulting on their loans, the stock market reflects a $240 billion loss. Firm after firm files for bankruptcy or sells themselves to bigger companies: Lehman Brothers, Merrill Lynch, and more. Corporations begin to yank their money out of money market funds, creating a huge spike in short-term interest rates. The Dow Jones Industrial Average falls 449 points.

The men at FrontPoint watch as the market falls, and within minutes they are up $10 million. Their seventy different bets on worldwide financial institutions are cashing in. In the midst of this, Danny Moses has a heart attack from the sheer chaos of the situation. Meanwhile, Cornwall Capital has quadrupled their capital, but are still too shocked at the downfall to celebrate. Burry, too, finds it hard to revel in his success as he wonders how people might view his financial strategy as morbid or distorted in some way. His investors have been more ungrateful for his strategy than he expected and it gives him one more reason to get out of money management. Even though he is more successful than most people who bet against the market, there is little to no recognition for his success.

EPILOGUE: EVERYTHING IS CORRELATED

Even though the fall has come and gone, the author explains that it takes a long time to change the American financial culture. This is simply because the things they had been doing wrong were being done wrong for such a long time, that it is all ingrained in the culture as being normal. Lewis traces some of the ideas that started the subprime crisis all the way back to the 1980s, suggesting that it will take even more than government intervention to clean up what Wall Street and these firms have done.

Even more disturbing, he points out, is the fact that most of the big players (both for and against the market) came out incredibly rich. The men at FrontPoint, Cornwall, and Scion all made tens of millions of dollars for themselves. But, people like Lippmann, Hubler and Wing Chau, who gambled with and lost billions of other's people money, came out of the crisis with millions of their own. The government stepped in to bail out Wall Street firms that had bankrupted themselves. This highlights his main point: the incentives on Wall Street are all wrong if people can get rich by making stupid decisions.

AFTERWORD

Michael Lewis provides a short afterword, explaining that this was the first of his novels that was not inherently comical. He admits that there are funny parts to the story, but he considers this to be a tragedy. He also explains how this novel legitimized him in a sense: people will now come up to him as if he were a money manager himself and ask for his advice. Even politicians approach him about the subject matter, and in some cases, do so over speaking to the men who actually lived the crisis for themselves. He suggests that him becoming an authority on this subject is merely because the government is now forced to clean up Wall Street, but it is completely impossible for any outsider to understand the machine without help. Therefore, without anyone else legitimate in Wall Street to trust, people turn to him.

ANALYSIS

This work offers an in depth look at the range of interesting people who bet against the subprime mortgage market and succeeded when it crashed. The author also explains, in depth, the catalysts behind the crash, the institutions and firms involved in setting it up, and how massive the downfall truly was.

A strength of the book is how it profiles a wide range of individuals who experienced the crash first hand. These characters put a human quality into the story of the Wall Street mortgage machine, and without them, the novel would likely be difficult for readers to swallow. There is a huge amount of factual information in this book, which is important to the credibility of the story, as well as for the reader to understand the full implications of what happened. However, due to this, as well as the copious amounts of financial jargon that becomes increasingly difficult for a layman to understand as the author reaches the depths of how the market crashed, the book is not easily accessible for the average reader. By including the stories of, and anecdotes from, these men who were able to find success in the housing market's failure, it adds an element of human interest for any reader who may begin to feel bogged down by the numbers.

This leads into a weakness of this book, as in it has a very specific audience. Once again, due to the vast amounts of technical language, even as Lewis does his best to explain the events as clearly as he can and with many colorful metaphors, it is easy for any reader lacking a financial background to get lost. To be fair, Lewis does mention several times how even the most experienced money manager or Wall Street investor finds confusion in the language and rules of the housing market. Yet, it still does not make for a light or easy read.

One of the foundational assumptions of this novel is that the reader is knowledgeable about the housing market crash in 2008. Lewis makes references to companies, news stories, and articles that were publicized at that time, and should be common knowledge for a reader who would care to pick up this kind of book. Even if a reader is lacking this priors knowledge, and has no experience in the financial or housing market worlds whatsoever, it is possible to find interesting points in his novel as his voice and ability to highlight human interest is what keeps the reader's attention.

While his main point is how the corruption and greed of Wall Street led to the collapse of the housing market, another issue that needs to be addressed is that these men who foresaw it— the good guys, essentially—also made a profit from the crisis. Lewis does portray some of the negative effects that these men experienced from their success, but it is not quite discussed or pointed out the irony that they were making money off the defaults of homeowners as well. Looked at in that light, how much more different are they than the villains that headed up the Wall Street banks and firms that created the loans in the first place?

The quality of research in this novel is impeccable as the author displays his credibility through first hand interviews with Eisman, Burry, and the others. His factual information is cited in the back of the novel and comes from many reputable sources. Lewis, being a financial reporter, understands the importance of citing sources and providing the reader with the exact quotes and words from his interviewees.

What the reader can take from the book is just how preventable the housing collapse truly was and also how to avoid being a victim of Wall Street greed. By learning what blinded consumers to participating in these loans in the first place, the reader can now see how to be vigilant against similar tricks that may be utilized by banks or other financial institutions in the future. It may not be possible for readers to have a hand in tearing down the corruption in Wall Street by reading a book, but it is possible for them to be alerted to their tricks in the hopes that it will make us smarter consumers.

Made in the USA
San Bernardino, CA
11 January 2017